Be Healthy Now!
Your Passport to Wellness

NUTRITION RESPONSE
TESTING^{SM}

by Paul J. Rosen, J.D., L.Ac., EAMP

Be Healthy Now!
Your Passport to Wellness
Copyright ©2011 Paul J. Rosen
Second Edition

Publishing by Warren Publishing, Inc.
Huntersville, North Carolina
www.warrenpublishing.net
ISBN: 978-1-886057-40-1

Printed in the United States of America

Welcome!

Name

_____

Date

_____

TABLE OF CONTENTS

DEDICATION

This book is dedicated to all of us, men, women and children alike, who are handling our most pressing health concerns by sticking to our guns in the knowledge that drugs and surgery are not the holy grail of healthcare. We are taking control of our own health by opening our minds to new approaches and being willing to make the necessary changes in and improve the quality of our lives using safe, natural and effective methods.

ACKNOWLEDGEMENTS

I am grateful to the following people who gave me life, saved my life, continue to sustain my life and make it possible for me to serve others in a way I could only have dreamed of. Gratitude is the reason to serve, and service is the means by which we are fulfilled and help others to fulfill themselves.

I want to thank my parents, Madalyn and Stanley Q; my teachers Swami Chetanananda, Rudi and Bhagawan Nityananda; Drs. Freddie Ulan, Bong Dal Kim and Richard Tan. There have been many others, too, who have been willing to share what they know in furtherance of my growth; you know who you are and I thank you.

Of course, if it weren't for the efforts of Cathy Brophy, my editor and publisher, the book would not have been completed. Thank you. Regarding copyediting, thank you Beth Hunter, Janeen Canfield, Angie Atkinson, Lisa Kolpeck and my wife.

Finally, to my wife Cheryl, whose love and companionship have made and continue to make it possible for me to do whatever I'm doing on our journey together. Thank you, my dearest darling!

Thanks~
P

PREFACE

Once upon a time, I lived my life eating Kellogg's Frosted Flakes, chocolate cake, and ice cream. And it was good. As a teenager I wanted to be healthy, so I added a multiple vitamin, changed my cereal to granola and continued to consume plenty of Coca-Cola.

As a young adult, I ate more fresh veggies but continued to eat the occasional chocolate chip cookie or brownie. And I couldn't see giving up my ice cream. I was certain that I was eating healthy, or at least healthier than most ~ wasn't I?

Fast forward to age 45. I found myself lying on the floor in an airport terminal with a heart that couldn't keep a rhythm. In other words, I crashed ~ my health, that is. As it turns out, not everyone crashes as hard as I did, but most everyone experiences signs of deterioration. You'll know you're deteriorating because you've got symptoms ~ any symptoms?

This is because disease is present when symptoms are present. Disease is the normal reaction to an abnormal environment ~ the physical body in this case. Disease is a silent process until it speaks with symptoms.

Most of us don't get serious about eating healthier until our health is challenged in a way that scares us. You say, "But I already eat healthy: whole grains, fruits and vegetables." But you add the daily power bar (a source of concentrated sweetener), corn or potato chips (saturated in rancid oils), that soy latte (full of sweeteners and powerful hormone stimulants) or a chocolate treat (likewise laden with sweeteners and often processing chemicals).

For most of us this is reality. And I hear it all the time. "Everyone does it, so it must be alright." "Without my treats, life isn't worth living." "How could I ever stop eating sugar when it's in everything?" "If I can't eat those things, what's left?" So what can you eat? We'll get to that in a bit.

These concerns are real and legitimate. How many people can even contemplate avoiding sugar? I know it was unimaginable to me. So I began where I could: reducing the number of times I ate ice cream from every night to every other night. At first, I felt deprived. I don't exactly know when it dawned on me, but I realized that the only thing I was being deprived of was my health.

Each and every one of you will have your own realization about what's most important for you. My purpose in writing this is to assisit your health coach to take you step-by-step as far as you're willing to go toward attaining the best health you're willing to accept. The information in this book is your key to attaining your best health ever.

You're probably reading this book because you've been evaluated by a qualified practitioner using Nutrition Response Testing and have made the move to become a patient. If so, your practitioner has all of the support staff, products and procedures in place to ensure your success. Learn all you can. There are articles, handouts and plenty of first-hand experience in the office because every staff member has his or her own health story to tell. Ask them!

If you have not been evaluated by a qualified Nutrition Response Testing practitioner, then your first step should be to find a qualified practitioner and get evaluated. Contact Ulan Nutritional Systems at 866-418-4801, and they will be delighted to find you such a practitioner. In the meantime, there are plenty of useful tips and life-changing information you can take advantage of right now. So please ~ read on.

WELCOME ABOARD

You're now a patient. Congratulations! You've chosen to take your health back and you're sure to get results. Just follow in the footsteps of thousands of others across this nation, including myself. Be sure to read and re-read this handbook. It's chock full of information, including the practical steps you'll take to transform the quality of your life. Remember, to change your life you are going to have to make changes in your lifestyle. AND to change your lifestyle, you've got to change your habits.

If you are feeling a bit overwhelmed, that's to be expected. Don't fret. The only way to get to the top of a mountain is to take a step at a time. Before you know it, the *new* you will begin to appear. And that's who you've been looking for.

A NUTRITIONAL HEALING PROGRAM DESIGNED ESPECIALLY FOR YOU

Probably one of the most confusing subjects when it comes to nutrition is diet. Which diet is the best? Is there a diet that fits everyone, or does everyone require a personalized diet? And, if everyone requires a personalized diet, is there a way to ensure you get it right?

Let's take the first question: which diet is the best? Quite simply, the one that works for you. "Works for you" means that you are symptom-free, emotionally balanced, sleeping well and full of vitality.

Is there a diet that fits everyone? So many people have written books proclaiming they've found the diet that really works. If you're like me, you have tried many of these without results. Why? Because what these folks have found is the diet that works really, really well **for them**. And if they're the enterprising type, they want to share it with everyone. Sure, others may see benefits, too. To know why, let's look at a key factor that all diets or diet plans share.

Despite the obvious commonalities (like food types), what they have in common is what's missing. I repeat, what they have in common is what they're missing or avoiding.

You see, each one of those diet proponents stopped eating something that they were eating before. It might have been an animal product, a grain or sugar. And it is what they stopped eating ~ the food substance that was overwhelming their bodies ~ that was the catalyst to regaining their health.

Conclusion, people are different and have different nutritional requirements. This is why I declare over and over in my book, *The Great Health Heist*, that you must discover who you are. Does your body work better with ingesting more or less animal, vegetable or mineral? Is there a dependable way to find out? Answer, yes!

That's where Nutrition Response Testing technology shines. And by following your individualized nutritional healing program, you're about to discover the power of "you."

WHERE DO I BEGIN ~ NOW WHAT?

You've gotten your nutritional supplements, your refrigerator page and a cheery congratulations from the staff. Now go home and take some time to re-read your personalized report of findings. That document is the culmination of decades worth of experience and will answer many questions and keep you on the path to wellness.

Do not stop taking any supplements unless directed by your nutrition practitioner. Likewise, do not stop taking prescription medications without the knowledge of your prescribing physician.

Keep your appointments unless there is an emergency. Weekly visits are extremely important to your success. After all, if you knew how to make this transition successfully by yourself, you would have done it already. If you do have to miss a visit, be sure to reschedule during the same week, if possible. You're here to learn and successfully transition to a new state of health.

Remember, communication is the key to understanding, and understanding is the key to progress. So communicate! Communicate your concerns and questions and, of course, your wins. After all, we're here to help.

If you haven't yet been introduced to Nutrition Response Testing, I urge you to learn more about it. It will change your life. But whether you are a patient or not, this booklet is designed to give you the tools you need to get your health back.

TAKING YOUR SUPPLEMENTS

Does it matter what brand of vitamin I use? After all, aren't all vitamins the same?

Yes, brand does matter when it comes to vitamins. And no, all vitamins are not created equal. Most over-the-counter brands are full of additives and foreign substances and who knows what else.

The supplements we recommend are used *because they work*. In the case of Standard Process, they've worked since 1928. In my book, *The Great Health Heist*, I go into detail about Standard Process and its founder, Dr. Royal Lee. But I will emphasize that all of their whole-food supplements are tended with great care from the farm to the bottle. They are inspected at least five times to be sure that what Dr. Lee intended to be contained in a supplement is actually there. Most of their products are organic, and when they cannot be, they are inspected, and any foreign substance or contaminants are eliminated. Furthermore, no genetically modified food is used.

Patients often ask, "Why must I take supplements three times a day? Isn't twice enough?" The purpose of spreading supplements throughout the day is to provide your body with high quality replacement parts in a timely manner. You place the most stress on your system during the day and use the most fuel.

The same reasoning applies to not skipping meals. If you needed ten gallons of gas to make a hundred-mile trip, you wouldn't put in just nine gallons. You'd either have to slow way down to stretch your fuel consumption or stop along the way. You might get there, but it would take you longer ~ or you might be on foot and without your vehicle.

Similarly, your body's thyroid or adrenal glands are already weakened due to poor eating habits and environmental influences. Failure to provide the proper fuel will cause them and you to have to slow down, resulting in fatigue or worse. The key to optimal health is to get the proper fuel in a timely manner.

Having said that, if you simply cannot manage to take your supplements three times a day, taking them morning and afternoon will do just fine. Divide your daily dosages into two portions as opposed to three. But, regardless of how often you take them, the ticket is to take them faithfully. They work better that way.

And if you have difficulty swallowing pills, alert your practitioner, and he or she will assist you in designing a strategy. Practitioners and office staff are experts at this stuff, and no question is a dumb question. Take advantage of the support that is offered.

Do I Continue To Take My Other Supplements?

Any supplements you were taking before beginning your nutritional healing program should be maintained unless and until your practitioner recommends otherwise. Prescription medications should also be maintained and modified only with your prescribing physician's knowledge.

You've Started Taking Your Supplements And Something Seems Wrong

One directive we mention during your initial report of findings is that if, when you begin to take the supplements, you feel worse or get sick for any reason, you should call the practitioner's office to schedule a visit.

Although you may not know why you're having difficulty, you may think a supplement is the reason for your discomfort. You've tested well for all the products recommended, but good products can make you feel bad if you're not regulating well.

The clinical phenomenon you're experiencing is a lack of regulation. In other words, your autonomic nervous system is going through some changes. These changes are part of the healing process (sometimes referred to as a healing crisis or turning point).

These turning points are positive in every respect except one ~ your discomfort. No one said change would be discomfort-free. But, when monitored by an expert during such times, you get a glimpse into the next phase of your program. You can stop taking the supplements if you like and simply pick up the phone and call or email the practitioner. But, whatever you do, don't panic. Relax ~ we've got your back.

FOOD DIARIES ~ FOLLOW THE BREAD CRUMBS

Food diaries have been identified by patients as one of the most important tools for a successful transformation to healthy eating. Not only are you asked to write down the foods you eat (amounts are optional) but also your water intake, sleep quality, number of bowel movements and any difficulties you may be experiencing.

The process of record keeping informs you of how you're doing and what you're eating. It also provides the practitioner with the "bread crumbs" to assist you in tracking down problems.

A stubborn problem that confounds many patients is a phenomenon called "cross-contamination." This occurs when foods like wheat, corn, soy, dairy or eggs are processed in the same facility. Many products have labels that say just this. I refer to them as "get out of jail free" cards. This is because, now that food sensitivities are widely acknowledged, corporate lawyers have devised these labels as disclaimers. (You've now been warned, so don't blame the cow for soggy cornflakes, so to speak).

Cross-contamination is often the culprit, although you're sure you haven't consumed any soy or corn, the practitioner tests and finds it is affecting your regulation. This can be confusing and frustrating. The testing is accurate. So stop and take a deep breath. Your practitioner is trained to help you sort this out.

Other cross-contaminations may be intentional, such as a product that uses a protein isolate (read the labels). A protein isolate is just that: a protein isolated from a food source like wheat, whey, soy or corn, for example. Whey is the result of removing fat and carbohydrate from milk, a process that may compromise its food value. Most products on the store shelf test poorly when muscle-tested. Be sure to bring in any protein supplements, protein bars, wheat-grass products ~ anything, really. Think of it this way: you've probably been ingesting these things for some time, and yet your level of health is not what you'd hoped.

Just by reading the product labels, you will not reveal all the tricks and traps set both intentionally and unintentionally by food producers. But fear not ~ this, too, will be sorted out at your follow-up visits.

GO THROUGH YOUR KITCHEN CABINETS ~ SURPRISE!

The next step is to go through your kitchen cabinets, reading the labels on your food items. You will be shocked at what you find. Place items that contain sweeteners, grains or other foods you may be sensitive to in a box, and either donate or trash them. For some of you, your cupboards will be all but bare. So it's off to the market!

But before you jump into the car, take a moment to do some meal planning. Below you'll find some recommendations.

Since many of us have grain sensitivities, we have chosen dishes that use few if any grains. The following selections will work for most of you. However, some of you may need to avoid fruit, dairy and/or eggs, as indicated in your report of findings. If this is true for you, be sure to ask your patient advocate what to use to replace these items in your diet. And remember, food sensitivities are not necessarily for a lifetime. The idea is to avoid these foods for as long as it takes your body to heal itself. By the way, be sure to ask your practitioner to test you periodically to see if you can begin eating a food you've been told to avoid.

WHAT DO I EAT FOR BREAKFAST?

Breakfast is the most confusing meal for people, especially for those who need to avoid grain, eggs and/or dairy. I recommend that you first set aside all your preconceived ideas about breakfast. Know that we have been trained to eat cereal and muffins for breakfast. And yet, many people have problems with grain. The fact that we associate grains with breakfast is just a habit, really. And, as was mentioned before, it's your eating habits that got you into trouble in the first place. So forming new habits is key to your successful transformation into a healthier and happier YOU.

Breakfast is important, but it's the one meal that is often skipped by many. Skipping the morning meal ~ or any other meal for that matter ~ results in depriving your body of essential fuel, leading you to reach for stimulants like coffee and sugar later in the day. Breakfast should consist of the same nutrient-dense foods as lunch and dinner: vegetables (minerals), high-quality protein, and good fats like butter, olive oil or coconut oil.

Whether you walk gingerly into the water or jump in, the question that arises now is, what are you going to eat ~ especially for breakfast? Since most people today are habitually driven to eat cereal, toast, muffins, pancakes and waffles for breakfast, I understand the shock of discovering that grains are a problem. (After all, I'm sensitive to grains, too ~ and, yes, it was a shock at first).

Changing your eating patterns will require a shift in your thinking. Did you ever notice that when you buy a new car or article of clothing you begin to see them everywhere? It's kind of funny. These things were always present. It's just your awareness that has changed.

This same phenomenon holds true for most transformations. Someone like your nutrition practitioner makes you aware of a solution to a problem (namely, your health) that you've been trying to solve for a long time. And, as it turns out, a significant piece of the puzzle is food sensitivity.

Not everybody has food sensitivities, but these days it's pretty common. I bet you know someone who is gluten-intolerant. Gluten intolerance is associated with wheat. What you may not have known is that sensitivities to other grain products like soy and corn are just as common and often overlooked.

Your practitioner is trained to identify food sensitivities. And if you are one of the many people found to have some, they can be challenging to manage. So, as in every other aspect of a transformation, my advice is to make the change at a speed you can manage. If you are sensitive to wheat and can't face the notion of giving up bread all at once, then at least switch to a healthier product ~ from white bread to whole grain, for example. Just remember: if you're not seeing improvements in your health at the speed you'd hoped for, your practitioner will up the gradient and recommend that you avoid the bread altogether for at least 90 days. If you like the results, you can decide whether or not to continue the avoidance.

Does it take a commitment to make the transition to other foods for breakfast? Yes! But transition is the key. And it's not nearly as hard as you might think. Here's how you do it. . .

Recognition: We eat things we are accustomed to. This is a habit. And habits are changeable. (If we make them, we can change them.) So what about this idea? All the foods you eat for lunch and dinner can be eaten for breakfast. This sounds strange, I know, but once you've experienced an improvement in your health, you'll be glad you made the changes and wonder why you hadn't done it earlier.

You could keep doing what you've always done but that would put you back where you were ~ or worse. Understanding this small bit of truth should inspire you to persevere. But what if you get off track? Lose your way? Cheat?

That's why we are here: for support. In a world fraught with a food supply that is chock full of traps and challenges, having the technology to test foods and food products enables you to identify offenders quickly and easily.

WHAT DO I COOK MY FOOD IN?

What do you cook in? Microwave, convection oven, aluminum pots, pots covered with a non-stick surface? Here's the scoop. . .

Microwave ovens, although convenient, have been shown to alter food chemistry in ways that adversely impact your blood, immune system and cholesterol balance. All cooking of food destroys vitamins, but studies in Europe and Russia reveal that microwaving is by far the most harmful. Fewer vitamins are lost when food is cooked at lower temperatures for longer periods of time, which is why "slow cookers" are often a good choice. However, it's tough to roast a chicken in a slow cooker, so your best choice of ovens are the convection, toaster or everyday range for baking and cooking these larger items.

The mainstream media in the United States has, unfortunately, done a good job of convincing us all that aluminum and non-stick surfaced pots and pans are perfectly safe. Nothing could be farther from the truth.

Aluminum atoms detach from the pan's surface during cooking and mix with your food. Aluminum has no place in your body in any amount. It can damage any body part, but especially your brain, thyroid, kidneys, lungs and liver.

As far as the safety of non-stick surfaces is concerned, plenty of research reveals that heat breaks these coatings down, releasing toxic fumes, including several which are cancer-causing. The material you cook in should be as stable as possible when heated. Ceramic, glass and porcelain-coated pots and pans are your best choices, followed by high-quality stainless steel.

Now that your cooking utensils are safe, let's move on to the wonders of water.

WATER, WATER EVERYWHERE ~ BUT HOW MUCH & WHAT TO DRINK

There are so many opinions regarding water. Some argue you should drink when you're thirsty. Others say, "No, that's too late ~ drink at least half your body weight every day." And some people champion the old "eight glasses a day."

What to do? Frankly, I was as confused as you until I began my own nutritional healing program. The answer is (you guessed it) to get tested! People's individual needs differ.

Just as with anything else, your body's need for water varies from day to day. There's a handy way to self-test to see if you're getting it right. My colleague, Dr. Joe Teff, shared this with me some time ago. Here's how it works:

Stand with your hands by your side for a minute or two. Without raising your arms, look at the inside surface of your bare wrists and notice that your veins bulge a bit. Now extend the arm with the most obviously bulging vein straight out in front of you and watch your wrist. If the bulging vein(s) remains bulged, it means you are drinking sufficient fluids. If the bulge flattens, it indicates you are not consuming enough fluid.

Fluids should be sipped and not gulped. Consuming a lot of fluid at once results in your body eliminating most of it because it has no time for assimilation. In other words, you'll have to urinate. So the best way to hydrate is slowly, over time. If you are training or exercising rigorously, ask your practitioner for additional tips about hydration.

I'm often asked what type of water is best. My answer: your water should be pure and without additives ~ no colors, vitamins, minerals, flavors or sweeteners.

What's not recommended? Drinking from the tap! It isn't safe because too many industrial chemicals are present. Pharmaceuticals as well as pesticides, herbicides and fungicides from farming have been found in over 85% of our nation's community water supplies. And let's not forget about chlorine and fluoride.

Despite the fact that chlorine does function to keep the flora and fauna to acceptable levels, fluoride is mass medication with questionable effect. In any event, both should be filtered out of the water you drink, cook and bathe in because of ill effects on your endocrine system ~ especially your thyroid.

Regarding the type of water filter and which model is best, simply ask your practitioner. Many filtration systems are available.

Finally, I caution you about trying to regulate your body's pH with specialty water. It is not the most effective way to do it and often creates more problems than it solves. Consuming large amounts of alkaline or acidic water is a great way to mess up your digestive system. Diet changes are much more effective. And as for distilled water, avoid it! It is a cooked product that acts as a de-mineralizer in your body. In any event, now that you are on a personalized nutritional healing program, you have all of this covered.

In summary, how much water to consume depends on individual needs. Test and monitor your wrists. Be sure your water is pure and without colors, vitamins, added minerals, flavors or sweeteners. At a minimum, it should be filtered and, if bottled, the best is artesian or spring water.

SUGAR & CONCENTRATED SWEETENERS ~ WORSE THAN YOU THOUGHT

If you ask anyone who is health-conscious whether they eat sugar, they will admit to eating some but not as much as most people do. So, how much sugar do you eat? Have you made any attempt to find out?

There was a time in my life when I couldn't contemplate giving up ice cream. But when confronted with a life-threatening condition, I found it was either give it up or get ready for "the big sleep." I simply wasn't ready for the latter, so I gave it up.

Fortunately, for many of you, your health isn't as challenged as mine was. And sugar avoidance may appear to you to be a deal-breaker. However, because you recognize your health isn't what you'd like it to be, how about taking the first step? Do as so many others have done: eliminate one cookie, one soft drink, one candy bar at a time.

And while you're contemplating that first step, let me share this bit of thought-provoking information: every human being has cancer cells (or at least the makings of them) running around in their body. When you want to be rid of a stray cat, one good way is to not feed it. Think of a cancer cell as that cat and sugar as its food.

A current technology used by Western Medicine to discover cancers in the body is Positron Emission Tomography or PET scan. This scan is accomplished by injecting the body with a radioactively tagged glucose (sugar) solution. The tissues most metabolically active, such as the brain or a cancer, absorb the solution faster. This is highlighted on the radiographic image. Do you see? Sugar enables cancer to thrive! Is that scary enough for you?

For optimal health, we have to avoid concentrated sweeteners including sugar, high-fructose corn syrup, fruit concentrates, agave syrup, maple syrup and honey at least until our bodies get healthier. Since the body is innately much smarter than you or me, we have to let it tell us when it's OK. And if you are diabetic, all sugars, grains and fruit are out of bounds.

DID YOU EVER WONDER WHAT IT FEELS LIKE TO EAT CORRECTLY?

What follows is the guide to knowing what it feels like to eat correctly. How are **you** doing?

If you answer yes to any of these questions after you eat a meal, **changes are required**:

- Are you physically full but still hungry or get hungry soon after you eat?
- Do you have cravings for sweets?
- Do you feel tired or too hyper?

- Do you find it difficult to focus mentally, are spacey or your mind races?
- Do you feel down, blue, apathetic or short-tempered?
- Do you experience any symptoms or aggravation of one of your chronic symptoms?

If you answer yes to these statements, then you're **getting it right**:

- You feel satisfied, not hungry or over-full.
- You have no sugar or other food cravings.
- You feel like your energy has been restored.
- Your mind is clear and sharp.
- You feel more emotionally balanced.
- You experience no symptoms and/or your chronic symptoms are improving.

By the time we're done I'm certain you'll be **getting it right!**

WHAT TO EAT ~ PLAN, SIMPLIFY & ORGANIZE

A Successful Transition As Seen Through Beth, My Office Manager's, Eyes

The following material is an example of how Beth goes about planning, simplifying and organizing her meals.

"Every three days," she says, "I prepare the staple foods I will use for meals. I always make a large pot of soup or stew, chop my fresh vegetables, prepare a high-quality protein (roasted or broiled meat), a faux granola snack (see recipe at end of this section) and a fresh salad around which I plan my meals."

Here is a copy of the FREE FOODS list. Use this to select the foods to make a grocery list. Note that, since you'll be reading every food label, shopping will take longer than it used to. Be prepared to be shocked at what you find. Eventually, however, you'll learn what foods support you, and shopping will once again be a snap.

FREE FOODS LIST

Vegetables (*if it says cooked, never eat raw ~ lightly steamed is okay*):

Alfalfa seeds (sprouted)
Arugula
Asparagus (cooked)
Bamboo shoots (cooked)
Beans, green (cooked)
Beet greens (cooked)
Broccoli (cooked)
Cabbage (cooked)
Carrots
Cauliflower (cooked)
Celeriac, celery root (cooked)
Celery
Chard, Swiss (cooked)
Collards (cooked)
Cucumber
Dandelion greens (cooked)
Eggplant (cooked)
Endive
Fennel bulb
Garlic
Hearts of palm
Jicama
Kale (cooked)
Lettuce, butterhead
Lettuce, green leaf
Lettuce, iceberg
Lettuce, red leaf

Lettuce, romaine
Mustard greens (cooked)
Mushrooms
Olives
Onions
Parsley
Peppers, green
Peppers, jalapeño
Peppers, red
Peppers, serrano
Pumpkin (cooked)
Purslane
Radicchio
Radishes
Rhubarb
Sauerkraut
Scallions, green onions
Spinach (cooked)
Squash, summer (cooked)
Squash, zucchini (cooked)
Tomatillos
Tomatoes
Tomato juice
Turnips (cooked)
Turnip greens (cooked)
Watercress

Fruit:
Apricots
Avocados
Blueberries

Prunes
Raspberries
Strawberries

<u>Nuts (*raw or dry-roasted*):</u>
Almonds
Cashews
Hazelnuts
Macadamia nuts
Peanuts
Pecans
Pistachios

<u>Meat and Seafood:</u>
Beef, lamb and poultry (free range,
    organic, chemical free)
Fish and caviar (fresh or wild caught)
Crab, lobster and shrimp

<u>Dairy (*raw is best*):</u>
Butter
Buttermilk
Cheese, cheddar
Cheese, cottage
Cheese, cream
Cheese, Edam
Cheese, feta
Cheese, goat
Cheese, Gouda
Cheese, ricotta (whole milk)
Cheese, Swiss

Half & half
Heavy cream
Milk, goat
Milk, whole
Yogurt, plain (whole milk)

Eggs (_organic/free range_):
Egg whites and yolks

Beverages:
Coffee (without cream or sugar)
Tea (without cream or sugar)
Water (spring or filtered)

Feel free to choose your own combination of foods from the Free Foods List. Beth records her "go to" shopping list:

Grocery List
- Celery
- Roasted Nut butter
- 1 Whole Chicken and/or Beef Roast
- Cold-pressed Olive Oil
- Sesame Oil
- Onions
- Carrots
- Red Peppers

- Cucumbers
- Chicken Broth
- Vegetable Broth
- Salsa
- Kalamata Olives
- Fresh Garlic
- Red Potatoes
- Kale
- Fresh Seasonal Vegetables
- Avocados
- Sea Salt
- Peppercorns
- Balsamic Vinegar
- Dry-roasted Pumpkin Seeds
- Coconut Cream Concentrate
- Stevia
- Romaine Lettuce
- Tomatoes
- Spring Water
- Lemon
- Organic Coconut Oil

"These are the essential items I have in my kitchen at all times. With these few foods, I'm able to create a multitude of delicious meals, including quick and easy ones for when I'm too busy to cook. I occasionally purchase other foods for special meals, but day-to-day I rely on these for most of my needs. You may notice I haven't selected eggs or dairy. That's only because I'm sensitive to both. I envy those of you who can partake of such joy. So think of me and be gentle with my soul whenever you eat cheese.", says Beth, my office manager.

It's important to be prepared in advance. This eliminates the temptation to eat quick foods that aren't good for you.

To begin the preparation, I recommend having on hand many sizes of airtight containers. These are what I store my cut up vegetables and leftovers in. Wash your celery (saving the leaves for soup), carrots, cucumbers and peppers. The amount of vegetables required is based on your personal appetite and how many people you're cooking for. For one person, I find the following quantities to be sufficient: 2 large carrots, 4 stalks of celery, 1 cucumber and 2 red peppers.

Snack food is always a must so, as promised, here's our delicious no-grain granola recipe. This consists of 1 part nut butter to 1 part coconut cream concentrate, with an equal amount of seeds or chopped nuts. After mixing all the ingredients, including sea salt and stevia for sweetener (only if necessary) to taste, place the mixture in a Ziploc bag and flatten. Then place the bag in the refrigerator. When the mixture has hardened, break it up into small bite-sized portions.

Convenient nutrient-dense dishes include soups and stews. Soup is a great way to get all you need in one bowl ~ fast. In fact, I recommend soup as your new "fast food." My favorite soup is quick and easy. I recommend you make this the old-fashioned way: on the stove in a big pot, although you could also use a slow-cooking crock pot.

I start with 2 cartons of chicken broth (use Imagine organic chicken broth or Pacific brand's organic Simply Stock because they contain no sugar), 2 cartons of vegetable broth (a brand with no added sugar), and 1 container of sugar-free salsa (I use Trader Joe's mild salsa). I chop 1 onion finely, the celery leaves, kale, and a couple cloves of fresh garlic to put in the pot. Now add your favorite chopped veggies and season to taste. If you want your soup to be a complete meal, add a whole chicken or 4 chicken parts to the pot. Let it cook until the meat appears to fall from the bones. Let it cool, and remove the meat from the bones.

Store in the refrigerator. (Note: Always let things cool before placing in plastic storage containers. And if you do put something hot in the fridge, leave the lid ajar to allow the steam to escape.)

This wholesome dish can be used for your breakfast every morning as well as your meal replacement for days when you don't have time to cook. Of course, if you don't like chicken soup, you can substitute turkey, fish, beef, pork, or lamb.

"I understand this is a major lifestyle change and want you to know there's hope."

During your transition into healthy eating, a helpful approach includes something I learned along the way: focus on what you can eat and not on what you can't. Remember, Beth's approach is one that works for her. You're free to improvise, keeping in mind that you avoid skipping meals, plan ahead and choose your foods from the FREE FOODS LIST. Eating fresh food is not only a necessity, it's delicious. Bon appétit!

Important Note: For a host of grain- and sugar-free recipes, simply go to our website, www.AcuNatural.com, where a selection of mouth-watering dishes await you. For even more ideas just Google grain-free cookbooks.

TO MARKET, TO MARKET

Once you've decided on your menu, go to the market and be sure to take your FREE FOODS list along. (This is the personalized list of foods I just provided above.) No sense putting more pressure on yourself to memorize it ~ that will come with time.

Once at the market, follow this rule of thumb: shop around the perimeter of the store. This is generally where you find fresh produce, the fish and meat counters and dairy products. The center aisles are where you can look for hard goods like sea salt, ready-made organic soup broths, canned tomatoes, laundry soap, and the like.

The perimeter of the store may also include some freshly prepared foods like rotisserie chickens, salad fixings and roasted vegetables. Here's where you might indulge your convenience gene. But always ask about spices that contain maltodextrin (from wheat) or protein isolate (from soy). READ LABELS, READ LABELS, READ LABELS!

KEEP IT FRESH! Fresh food provides nutrient-rich sources of vitamins and minerals our bodies need to restore and repair themselves. And always consider eating organic. Why is organic better?

First, there are no synthetic or man-made chemicals such as herbicides, pesticides or fungicides used in the process of growing or storing the food. By the way, that doesn't mean that organically grown crops are free of pesticides. It just means the pesticides are not synthetic. So always be sure to wash all raw produce.

Second, according to the USDA, "organic food is produced by farmers who emphasize the use of renewable resources and the conservation of soil and water to enhance environmental quality for future generations. Organic meat, poultry, egg, and dairy products come from animals that are given no antibiotics or growth hormones. Organic food is produced without using most conventional pesticides; petroleum-based fertilizers, or sewage sludge based fertilizers; bioengineering or ionizing radiation."

Finally, speaking of soil, no one wants to pay for something that they're not getting or at least getting less of what they want. Food grown in commercial soil versus organic soil contains fewer minerals (calcium, magnesium, potassium) and trace elements (boron, manganese, iron, copper and cobalt), all factors critical to good health. Healthy soil means healthy crops. And healthy crops mean a healthier you.

Once you start preparing your own food, you'll eat out less often, which saves money. The same is true for eating fewer packaged, processed goods, since we pay 30-40% more for them because all that packaging costs money. Many people who thought organic nuts, fruits and vegetables were too expensive have been able to buy them based on the savings above. If buying organic still seems too expensive, you can still eat fresh, but be sure to wash your produce thoroughly.

Food for thought: Janelle Sorensen, a senior writer and health consultant for the nonprofit organization Healthy Child Healthy World, wrote in an article published in July 2009 that the FDA admits that over 75% of processed food consumed in the U.S. is genetically modified (GM). Moreover, in its inimitably shortsighted wisdom, the FDA does not require that this food be labeled GM. So you've probably been eating genetically modified food every day for some time. Corn and soy are just two foods that are GM.

"Reality is that the FDA has absolutely no genetically modified organism (GMO) safety testing requirements, and GM ingredients are ubiquitous in prepared foods. Unless a processed food contains only organic ingredients, it is highly likely to contain GM ingredients. The 'research' that supports GMO safety is voluntarily provided by companies on their own GM crops and has been described by critics as 'meticulously designed to avoid finding problems.'

"But 44,000 FDA internal documents later made public as a result of a lawsuit revealed problems. The overwhelming consensus among the FDA's scientists was that GM foods were substantively different, so different that their consumption might result in unpredictable and hard-to-detect allergens, toxins, new diseases and nutritional problems. Agency scientists urged superiors to require long-term studies but were not only ignored, their statements about possible negative effects of GMOs were progressively deleted from FDA policy statement drafts."

Sorensen goes on to write: "According to Jeffrey Smith, author of *Seeds of Deception*, in one of the first studies in the early 1990s, rats were fed GM tomatoes. Actually, they refused to eat them, so they had to be force fed. And, rats aren't the only animals who've declined a snack of GMOs. Smith says 'eyewitness reports from all over North America describe how several types of animals, when given a choice, avoided eating GM food. These included cows, pigs, elk, deer, raccoons, squirrels, rats and mice. What do they know that people don't?"

Genetically modifying food involves, among other things, inserting genes to make the plant or animal pesticide-resistant. This means that they make their own pesticides. Research has shown that, when you ingest these foods, the friendly bacteria in your own stomach are altered and begin to churn out micro-amounts of the pesticide. That can't be a good thing.

Think about this information for a moment and then weigh the extra cost for organic foods versus the potential health risks posed by commercial foods. It could be money well spent.

And by the way, herbs are drugs ~ not pharmaceutical-grade but drugs, nonetheless.

This means they impact your autonomic nervous system (ANS) and can interfere with your regulation. Not all foods are supportive for all people. You are an individual with individual needs. Remember this! So bring your herbs in to be muscle-tested on you. This includes herbal teas and black, green or white teas ~ even if they are organic.

HOME AGAIN, HOME AGAIN

With your groceries in hand, prepare to wow the family. That goes for you men as well as you women.

One concern I hear a lot about is sugar cravings. "I've tried to avoid sugar but it's just too much." Ah, the words of a true addict. By eating nutrient-dense foods, including some animal protein and high quality fats, your taste buds will be reborn. In fact, one of the most pleasant surprises many patients experience is how the sugar cravings melt away.

By the way, natural sugar is in all fresh food ~ so don't get confused. The sugars we all must learn to avoid are ADDED PROCESSED SWEETENERS. If you need help identifying these, simply ask the staff.

Why do your cravings melt away? Because nutrient-dense food provides the body with the proper nutrition, while sugar and concentrated sweeteners deprive it of the same. And, since your taste buds are reborn every ten days or so, doing the right things gets results pretty quickly.

RESTAURANTS ~ TO EAT OUT OR NOT TO EAT OUT

Many people eat out often ~ that old convenience gene again. Others simply need a break from the routine of cooking. Eating out, however, can be a challenge.

When you do eat out, your rule of thumb is, no soups, no sauces, no salad dressings. Soups and sauces are often thickened with grains like cornstarch or wheat flour and may contain sweeteners. Salad dressings are rarely made without concentrated sweeteners. (Request olive oil and balsamic vinegar on the side to dress your own salad.) The awakening for most patients is finding sugar in everything. So be aware and don't hesitate to ask your waitress/waiter to find out ingredients.

Restaurants are in business to make money. Cheap food means cheap ingredients. Unfortunately, expensive food also can contain cheap ingredients. By "cheap ingredients" I mean those that are processed or commercially grown using pesticides, herbicides or fungicides. They may contain fillers like maltodextrin (a grain product) and sugar. This is especially true for spice mixes like Mexican, Thai, Italian, Indian and Chinese blends. If you like to cook with these spice blends, bring them to your practitioner for testing. It's better to be safe than sorry.

The next thing to consider when eating out is to select a restaurant where you can successfully avoid your food sensitivities. If you are sensitive to corn, then going to a Mexican restaurant is a sure loser. Likewise, if you are sensitive to soy and select a Chinese or Thai restaurant, you will be in trouble. What you are looking for is a restaurant that serves fresh food in simple ways, salads, grilled or roasted meat, poultry or fish, vegetables, both raw and cooked and perhaps a freshly baked potato or rice if you are allowed them in your nutritional healing program.

Now that you've selected your restaurant, prepare to order. When the waitress/waiter arrives, tell them you need their help, using an appreciative tone. You have food sensitivities, and would they please be sure that any food you order does not touch or contain, for example, any grains or concentrated sweeteners.

If they look at you as though you have two heads, simply get up and leave. It would be a sure sign that you'll regret it if you stay. I've never had that happen, and I have successfully navigated restaurants and enjoyed the meal and company. You can, too. Bon appétit!

FRIENDS & FAMILY GATHERINGS CAN BE A CHALLENGE

What about eating at a friend's or family member's home? This can present the biggest problem for most of you. It can be quite awkward to inform your hosts that you currently have some restrictions in your food choices. But, if you are truly committed to yourself, you will do just that.

You might be surprised at how accommodating your friends will be just so you all can enjoy each other's company. And if you're sitting there after dinner with a headache or stomachache because you ate some foods you should have avoided, you'll not be the best of company.

Beyond that, if you're enthusiastic about your new dietary choices, you may even offer to bring a dish over for them to enjoy. Truthfully, whenever there is an alternative dish prepared with fresh ingredients, it often disappears before the others do. It's happened to me many times.

Family gatherings are another story. Sometimes mothers and grandmothers are hurt if you don't eat what they've prepared "because I made it just for you, Dear." Depending on your relationship, you may feel forced to suffer the consequences.

Having grown up in a Jewish household, I know about that sort of thing. But I decided long ago that life has plenty of suffering without any input from me ~ so why do it to myself? It's your call, of course. Just don't be surprised if, at your next follow-up visit, your practitioner finds that you are not regulating and asks you to re-confirm your expectations for better health ~ with a smile, of course, and a gentle nudge back on track.

Falling off the wagon, so to speak, will happen and is absolutely no problem. Simply get back on the path, put one foot in front of the other, and the mountaintop will be that much closer. Better health is not an IF ~ it's a WHEN.

TRAVELIN' ALONG

Do you travel often? I did; teaching practitioners throughout the Western United States. The key to maintaining your food program on the road is PLANNING.

Onboard the plane, I always carry food: cut up fresh or cooked veggies, olives, cold chicken or beef, lots of nuts. And I always buy a bottle of spring water on the way to the gate after exiting security. (The water served on planes is normally not the best.)

In my checked bag, I pack a container of manageable breakfast foods, snacks (like nuts and seeds) and supplements.

I check this bag to avoid any conflict during flight check-in. I've never had any problem bringing supplements on board an aircraft, but since I check a bag with foods, I just throw in the supplements along with them (except for those I will take during the flight).

If you are treating active scars and have your own laser light, you can take the light on board or pack it. I've never had a problem either way.

When I arrive at my destination, I locate the nearest health food store (if one is available) or grocery store (if one is not). I buy bottled water, a few fresh vegetables and some nut butter (peanut, almond or cashew), roasted chicken and some organic eggs. Most hotels will supply you with a small refrigerator if you request one because of dietary restrictions.

If you are traveling by car, then it's a breeze. You can pack a cooler with just about everything you'll need. And speaking of cars, always have a bottle of water and some nuts or nut butter available in case you get hungry while running errands. It's all about PLANNING! It doesn't take long and it ensures success.

PERSONAL HYGIENE ~ LOOKIN' GOOD BUT FEELIN' BAD?

Skin, Hair, Underarm Care And Cosmetics

"No cosmetic looks as good as HEALTHY SKIN." So says my friend and office manager, Beth. And she's got lovely skin!

Cross-contamination is a problem with cosmetics, hair and skincare products, soaps and detergents. I refer you back to the protein isolate discussion and remind you to read the labels. If you see a long list with ingredients you cannot pronounce, you definitely do not want it on your body. But first, you deserve to know a bit about the industry that makes these products.

The more you look, the more you see. As a self-designated change agent for health and healthcare, I am always on the lookout for dis- and misinformation, and I've noticed a lot lately.

While I was researching for this book, I came across the title *Toxic Beauty*, a book written by Dr. Samuel Epstein, who is a well-known expert in the field of cancer causing agents. Wow, this book is an eye opener. What jumped out at me?

There are over 10,500 personal beauty and cosmetic products available in North America. Ninety-nine percent of them have at least one ingredient that has never been tested for safety.

Now get this: The phrase "For professional use only" that we find on so-called higher quality beauty products allows the manufacturer to remove harmful chemicals from the LABEL ~ not the product, just the label. In addition, the terms "hypoallergenic," "allergy-free," or "safe for sensitive skin" can be placed on products without actual testing, and neither the FDA nor any other regulating body even requires the companies to prove their claims. Finally, unless they are intentionally placed in the product, harmful chemicals do not have to be listed.

Consumer Reports revealed in a November 2, 2009, article by Naomi Starkman, a food policy media consultant, that canned foods contain many more times the legal amount of Bisphenol A (BPA). BPA is a chemical used to line clear plastic food containers and cans and is linked to a wide array of health issues, including reproductive abnormalities, heightened risk of breast and prostate cancers, diabetes, and heart disease. Despite the danger, the FDA is still looking into the findings.

Now that we've established that we're left almost completely in the dark with respect to product safety and their effects on our health, here's why we should care. . .

Our skin is a vital organ of our body. Like a lung, heart or kidney, it has specific functions. In fact, from the standpoint of function, skin is often referred to as the third kidney. For example, both excrete liquid to eliminate waste. And the health of the kidney is reflected in the health of the skin. This means that if you have skin problems like psoriasis, acne or eczema, we must look to your kidneys as part of the strategy to clean things up.

Skin is also absorbent. Therefore anything we put on our skins soaks into our bodies to some degree. Deodorants often contain aluminum to stop perspiration and propylene glycol as a drying agent. Aluminum has been associated with many chronic health conditions. In my clinic, chronic bladder problems, MS, Alzheimer's and Parkinson's patients all muscle-test for heavy metals, including aluminum.

Propylene glycol is the main ingredient of anti-freeze ~ yes, the colored liquid we pour into our car radiators to prevent engine freeze-up. The material safety data sheet warns users to avoid skin contact with propylene glycol as this strong skin irritant can cause liver abnormalities and kidney damage.

Women who have hormone imbalances should look largely to cosmetics and beauty products as a major factor. This is because many of them contain estrogenic chemicals, essences or soy. And soy is full of estrogenic chemicals.

These chemicals cause hormone imbalance. Result: your face creams, lipsticks and body lotions (with their dangerous chemicals) are undermining the function of your thyroid, ovaries and adrenal glands. If you are taking hormones do you have menstrual irregularities or stubborn menopausal symptoms? Do you battle irritability, blue moods, dry skin, thinning hair and fatigue? Any one or more of these symptoms can be the result of self-poisoning over days, months or years. In other words, you could be doing it to yourself and not even know it.

I don't know about you, but that really riles my bile. Organizations that should be protecting our interests, that we fund to protect our interests, are not. This leaves us to fend for ourselves, and the best weapon for our defense is knowledge. So it behooves each of us to become aware. READ THE LABELS!

All of this should send the ordinary human being scurrying to use natural products. Unfortunately, many natural products still contain unwanted ingredients like alcohol. They also contain herbs or herbal essences that can cause problems for the autonomic nervous system's regulation. (Remember our earlier discussion that herbs are drugs.) For example, lavender is known to stress the thyroid gland. The same is true for peppermint and other mints.

So what to do? First, if you agree that environmentally safe products offer you the best chance of avoiding contamination from soy and chemicals then refer to the website **ewg.org**. With a few strokes of the keyboard you can type in any maker's product for it's rating on the 'green scale'.

Remember, this is not about 'tree hugging green', although personally I'm all for it. This is about knowledge you can rely on to avoid contact with unwanted ingredients that undermine your health.

Once you've obtained the product, bring it to your Nutrition Response Testing practitioner who will muscle test you. They'll help you find out which products are truly your friends and which are not.

Healthy Skin Is In

And skin care? Tropical Tradition's coconut oil, skin cream, moisture lotion and lip balm work wonders. Another patient favorite is organic virgin olive oil, the emollient of the Egyptians, Greeks and Italians. In fact, I've been shaving with olive oil for years, and my skin has never been better. Oh, and my wife likes Dr. Bronner's Magic unscented organic lip balm.

What about soap? There is the new product line on the block ~ AcuNaturals Organics. Designed especially for those who are sensitive to fragrances and chemicals. And yes, Tropical Traditions, who has a pump foam soap made from ~ you guessed it ~ coconut. Both are fabulous.

By now you must think I own stock in Tropical Traditions. Trust me, I don't, and there are a number of other organic coconut products in the marketplace, but they don't seem to muscle-test well. I'm speculating, but I believe it's the way they are processed. But no matter which product you choose, be sure it muscle-tests well. And that goes for all products that come in contact with your body.

Speaking of body contact, don't overlook your dish soap and laundry detergent. The most consistent product to muscle-test well is ECOVER, an all-natural product that I've never found to be cross-contaminated with soy, the most common protein isolate in soaps. (Monsanto, the agricultural bio-tech conglomerate, and its pals have to do something with all that genetically modified soy they're touting.)

Hair Care

What about hair care products? We have that covered, too. Tropical Traditions has a coconut bar soap and a liquid pump soap liked by both men and women. For hair that is short, long, curly or straight, it works beautifully. (And a dab of their coconut oil as a leave-in conditioner is great.)

Several other products to consider are Dr. Bronner's Pure Almond Castille Soap and Jason's Natural Apricot Soap and Conditioner. You may find Dr. Bronner's Soaps at www.drbronner.com and Jason's Natural Apricot Soap and Conditioner at www.jason-personalcare.com.

Please keep in mind that even though these products are labeled pure or natural or even organic, they may not be right for your treatment program. Before you use any commercial product, have your practitioner use muscle testing to determine what is best for your overall health in regard to your treatment program. Your practitioner may have some other product suggestions, as well.

Antiperspirant Alternatives

For an antiperspirant, we find that applying organic coconut oil (made by Tropical Traditions) satisfies most of us. Some people, however, prefer using a solution of baking soda and water. And others use white vinegar and love it. If the baking soda or vinegar irritates your skin, try the other. In the case of baking soda, irritation indicates your skin is too alkaline. If vinegar irritates your skin, it indicates your skin is too acidic. Simple chemistry!

Finally, for those extra odiferous days, try 'Pit Stop', the men's version only. Just 'google pit stop' for the nearest retailer.

Granted, these options may leave you with some body odor, but most of my patients enthusiastically endorse these natural alternatives. By the way, the thyroid, liver, kidneys and bowels are the body's odor generators. As these organs get healthier, your body odor will noticeably lessen.

After poisoning myself with aluminum and propylene glycol (two ingredients found in antiperspirants) for decades, as many others have, I was amazed at how well coconut oil works. Several other product suggestions are Jason's Natural Cosmetics and Natures Gate. Remember when using a commercial product, have your practitioner use the muscle-testing to determine one that supports your overall health improvement program.

And for those of you who are concerned about offending others, contemplate this: the science of pheromones reminds us that our own essence can attract the perfect mate or keep you with the one you have. I can't tell you how often I hear people tell me they like the natural fragrance of their mate and how much they miss it when it's gone.

Beautification

Makeup is a stickier wicket. Here, I remind you to visit ewg.org for the 'green rating'. A brand to check out is Alima. Your safest bet is to use products that are loose mineral powders without other additives.

Metals are what give mineral products their color and you may or may not test well for the silvers, greens, pinks, purples or whatever. To be on the safe side, before you put it on your face have it tested by your practitioner.

Eyeliner, eye shadow and lip color are the hardest to find without some chemicals. Because European regulations are more strict than ours, their products do not contain such things as arsenic, lead, mercury, parabens and other known cancer causing agents.

For eyeliner and eye shadow use the mineral makeup suggested above. For lip color you'll need a lip liner and lip balm. For lip liner check out Lancome and for lip balm look for Dr, Bronner's Naked or Tropical Traditions unscented coconut. Check out WildernessFamilyNaturals.com. for mascara. But be sure to have them all tested before using them. Shortly, you will find yourself adept at reading ingredient lists and eliminating problem products.

Sunscreen

I'm often asked to recommend a sunscreen product. So let's talk about the sun and its effect on your body.

You're quite familiar with all the news about the importance of Vitamin D and its links to cardio-vascular health (high blood pressure), diabetes, obesity, fibromyalgia, mental emotional health (depression, schizophrenia, Alzheimer's and dementia), immune health (colds, flu, asthma), fertility, digestive health (Crohn's disease, IBD), osteoporosis, cancer (melanoma), MS ~ and the list keeps growing. Vitamin D appears to be connected to almost everything in the body from the bones to the brain.

Your body is capable of manufacturing its own Vitamin D, but only exposure to the sun can accomplish this. So, although sunscreens may protect you in the short term, they prevent this magical phenomenon from occurring. This leaves you susceptible to deficiencies. So, what's the plan?

Protection is necessary, especially for fair-skinned people who get little sun during most of the year and travel to their tropical paradise only to render themselves like a boar on a barbecue spit. So, the **first line of protection is to wear sun-protective**

clothing. Google "sun-protective clothing" and a selection of websites will appear.

Second, avoid sunscreen products that contain synthetic ingredients such as chemical fragrances, parabens and nano-particles. Titanium and zinc oxides are the "heavy lifters" in any product ~ the higher the SPF rating the higher the concentration of each of these. Other ingredients include oils such as coconut, sunflower, eucalyptus, jojoba and shea butter, as well as moisturizers like glycerine and preservatives such as synthetic vitamin E (d-alpha tocopherol).

Finally, be sure to have your practitioner test you for deficiencies in calcium, Vitamin D, Vitamin C and EFA's (essential fatty acids). These are critical components needed to ensure, among other things, activation of melanin. Melanin is responsible for your skin color and tanning. Supplementation may be recommended, including the Standard Process product Cataplex F Perles.

You can see that, with all these ingredients, just one may not muscle-test well, rendering the product less than optimum. So, in the case of sunscreens, the goal is to find the least onerous, since protection is recommended.

As a melanoma survivor myself, I choose clothing over sunscreens. I do not shy away from the sun. I raise dahlias, walk as often as I can, and love the outdoors. There is nothing like the sun to lift your spirits!

Don't Bug Me

Bug repellants come up almost as often as sunscreen products. All I can say is: CLOTHING, CLOTHING, CLOTHING.

Chemical products are simply out of the question. For example, DEET has been shown to melt plastic bags and fishing line. And, it was originally designed as a pesticide. Need I say more?

So what natural ingredients have been shown to repel mosquitoes and other pests? The most common are citronella, lemon grass oil, peppermint oil and vanillin. Again, any one of these may fail to muscle-test well, so beware.

As a general note, the products I have shared have muscle-tested well for more than 95% of those evaluated. BUT be sure to have your practitioner test them on you before using them. After all, the key to successfully restoring your health is to know precisely what your body has to say. And that's the beauty of Nutrition Response

Testing ~ its ability to reveal your individualized needs with laser-like accuracy.

CLEANING TIPS FROM "THE CANARY IN THE MINE"

My wife is what I like to call "the canary in the mine" when it comes to chemical sensitivities. To complicate matters, she's a cleaner (things really must be clean, if you know what I mean). The following are some tips that have met both her chemical issues and "neat freak" nature.

For cleaning products, there is nothing like Dr. Bronner's Almond-Hemp soap. You can use it to clean the floors, walls, bathrooms and more. And that includes hand-washing of delicate clothing ~ including her sweaters and pashmina shawls.

OxoBrite, as well as a product called It Works!, can add a bit of extra luster for your toilets, tubs and showers. OxoBrite's hand-sized white pads are water-activated and can be found at www.QVC.com. With a bit of water and "elbow grease," they remove built-up soap scum like magic.

For dusting, micro-fiber cloths and water are efficient and effective. And for the bacteria-phobic types, a steam cleaner is more than sufficient to eliminate the microscopic bugs of your nightmares. There is nothing like boiling water to do the trick. Both upright and hand-held steamers are available, so do a quick web search and you'll find a product that will suit your needs. (My wife uses Haan-brand steamers from www.QVC.com.)

FAQ'S
(If You Don't Ask You'll Never Know!)

Why You Might Feel Worse After Starting The Program

It is not unusual to experience either an aggravation of symptoms, or some new ones, when you begin your program or throughout the process of healing. Should you find yourself in this situation and are concerned, be sure to contact the clinic staff and make an appointment to be seen by your practitioner. The solution is at hand.

For example, if you have an active scar, it may need intensive treatment. So instead of getting light treatments only once a week, several treatments a week may be necessary. In special cases, your practitioner might recommend that you purchase your own laser light for home treatment. My wife, for instance, has a scar on her lip that she lasers once or twice a day, putting a smile back on her face in the process.

Regarding dietary changes, eliminating foods like sugar may result in withdrawal symptoms. Minor changes in your program will enable you to cruise by this phase. And speak to your clinic's patient advocate. We are trained and enthusiastic in our desire to help you through any rocky patches. After all, we've all been there!

Finally, you may be reacting to the new supplements you are taking. And this is because they are good for you. The supplements we use are derived from whole live foods. I repeat, whole live foods. Since your body is accustomed to processing mostly dead (processed) or fractionated foods, it may not be ready to handle live nutrient-dense substances. Once again, minor changes will be made in your program if indicated, and off you go.

Handling these atypical situations is routine for us ~ and they are always temporary. Remember, if your practitioner felt your case wasn't appropriate for Nutrition Response Testing, he or she would have said so at the outset. You agreed that change is what you needed to regain your health. And changes, while good, are not always symptom-free.

What Does "Regulation" Or "Regulating" Mean?

"Regulating" is a term we use to describe a body that is open to healing. You may recall that, in your initial evaluation, while using your arm to resist pressure, your practitioner placed the palm of her or his hand over your naval and asked you to "match the pressure." In this part of the evaluation, a normal sign was a weak muscle ~ your arm going down. In other words, a weakness here was a good sign. It meant your body was regulating.

What Does "Blocking" Mean?

When the autonomic nervous system (ANS) is stressed, it can be prevented from regulating specific organs or glands normally. When this happens, I use the term "blocked" or "blocking" to describe your condition. During the muscle test, if you experience a strong arm muscle when I place my hand over your ears, mouth, navel or hands, then your ANS's ability to regulate is blocked.

If your body is in this state, you may not see a change in your symptoms, or you may find a new symptom that hangs around, or you may just feel weak or experience fatigue. This condition will also weaken your immune system, making you susceptible to colds or flu. Think of it this way: how well can a bicycle wheel work with a stick stuck in the spokes? Our mission is to remove any impediments to your body's natural healing mechanisms.

When blocking occurs, it is important to identify the stressors or barriers to healing. These barriers include food sensitivities; immune challenges; chemical sensitivities, such as to formaldehyde, food dyes, colors and preservatives; metal sensitivities, such as to aluminum, mercury or lead; and external body scars. More on these barriers in sections to follow.

Once your barriers are identified, your practitioner will provide the solution in the form of a supplement, light treatment (in the case of an active scar), or other recommendation if needed. These actions restore normal regulation and progress toward better health resumes.

What Does "Switching" Mean?

As in the case of blocking, switching can occur when the ANS is under stress. Simply put, switching describes a condition of "going back and forth," "up and down," or "on and off." (Think of a light switch that turns a light on and off.)

During the muscle test, if you experience a weak muscle after you've placed your thumb and pinkie together on one hand with your eyes open or closed, then you are switched. In some cases, a state of switching exists at a deeper level of disturbance. In this situation, I check the strength of your muscle in one of many positions. For example, I will have you place a finger of one hand on your chin and a finger of your other hand on your navel. (My assistant Beth and I call this process of placing you in various positions "nutritional twister.")

Again, if switching occurs, you may experience "roller-coastering," (for instance, your symptoms improve and then worsen, or your energy rises and falls). Another phenomenon is the "opposite reaction." Examples of this are having an unpleasant reaction to a supplement you've tested well for or gaining weight on a diet despite exercise. In both cases one would have expected the opposite reaction. When switching occurs, it is important to identify the stressor(s). Once identified, your practitioner will provide the appropriate supplement (or light treatment in the case of a reactivated scar). This action restores normal regulation, and progress toward better health resumes.

How Do Scars Affect My Health?

Simple answer: a scar on the surface of your body can interfere with the normal regulation of the ANS. This interference prevents the body from healing. It can be the "missing piece" that, when handled, results in miraculous symptomatic relief. Therefore, scars are considered one of the key stressors. Let's take a closer look.

The ANS has two regulators, sympathetic and parasympathetic. You may have heard the phrases "fight or flight" and "relaxation response." The first of these refers to the sympathetic regulator while the second refers to the parasympathetic regulator.

The sympathetic regulator consists of a dense network of nerve fibers that are deployed over your entire body ~ like a silk stocking. When you cut your skin, you damage this stocking. When the skin heals, the nerve fibers simply do not knit together exactly the way they were before. (Imagine repairing a torn silk stocking.) The result is a potential for intermittent disruption in your nervous system, a disruption that can interfere with the normal regulation of your autonomic nervous system.

For a greater ease of understanding, metaphors may be useful. Think of a scar as either a capacitor or a circuit breaker. Both are electrical devices. A capacitor accumulates electrical potential. This potential needs to be regulated, or a surge of electrical energy will be released and create interference or disruption. Scars can act like capacitors but without regulation. Thus, they can create intermittent disruption of normal ANS regulation.

A circuit breaker is a switch on an electrical panel that can "pop off" when there is a surge of electricity and prevent potential damage. However, without electricity flowing through the circuit, normal operation of electrical devices ceases. Scars appear to "pop off" like a circuit breaker, thus disrupting normal regulation of the ANS. These are only metaphors, but they give you a good idea of what's happening. Whichever metaphor works best for you (capacitor or circuit breaker), a scar can be a key stressor that can cause intermittent interference with, or disruption, of normal ANS regulation.

When this condition is identified, applying wheat germ oil or sesame oil to the scar before treating it with a hand-held cold laser should deactivate the scar and eliminate the interference.

If You Don't Treat Your Scar, You Won't Go Far.

Scars are treated using a cold hand-held laser light held over the scar for three or four minutes. In addition, you should apply wheat germ or sesame seed oil to the scar on a daily basis, rubbing it in completely so as not to stain your clothes. Both treatments are designed to restore the flow of blood, nerves and body fluid through the scar tissue and re-establish normal regulation.

Some people notice the scar tissue disappearing over time. This goes for old, as well as new scars. In many instances, chronic pain and other symptoms disappear with the use of these techniques. Scars are just as important as the other barriers to healing. They must be actively treated in order to restore proper regulation ~ the key to getting well. This is why you'll often hear me say, "If you don't treat your scar, you won't go far."

How Long Must I Treat My Scars?

Some scars remain a potential cause of trouble for the ANS. Immune stressors like bacteria or parasites can adversely affect a scar. Likewise, an overly dense mass of fibrous tissue can be difficult for the laser to penetrate. In such situations, treatment using the oils and laser light may not be enough to permanently correct the condition.

Instead we might recommend applying specific products like Systemic Formula's Bactrex, Virox or Renovator to the scar's surface before using the laser light. For the toughest cases, a qualified practitioner might inject solutions of procaine or lidocaine to the periphery of the scar.

How Did I Get Food Sensitivities?

This is a complicated topic for which there is no simple answer. To begin, some of us come into this world with less than our fair share of digestive or metabolic enzymes (metabolic meaning "change" or "to change"). In our bodies, metabolism occurs to put substances together (like proteins, fats and carbohydrates) to form tissue. Metabolism also breaks things apart, like turning food into the proteins, fats and carbohydrates that provide the bio-energy needed to run our body's systems.

If we are missing specific enzymes to handle grains, eggs or dairy, the incomplete breakdown (metabolism) of these foods will result in larger than normal particulates that can attract the attention of our immune system. These larger than normal particulates may settle in the joints, for example, and cause the immune system to attack our joints, resulting in arthritis. These particulates may settle in the intestines, resulting in a similar attack causing IBD or celiac disease. These same particulates may create similar problems for other organs or glands and create a host of common symptoms.

Most of us eat highly processed or refined foods that overburden our metabolic enzyme bank. Each of us comes into the world with a limited bank or store of enzymes that we get to use any way we want. For instance, we can digest doughnuts and Dairy Queen or vegetables and fruits. Unlike highly refined foods, however, whole foods come with their own enzymes to aid digestion. This naturally eases the burden on our body's store of enzymes. In other words, by eating whole foods we can go farther on the enzymes we received at birth as our genetic share.

In an earlier section, I talked about genetically modified foods and the dangers they pose. It's worth mentioning again that the foreign genetic material that provides the plant's resistance to pesticides has been shown to co-opt the friendly bacteria in our gut. This means that your gut continues to make these pesticide poisons long after the food has been evacuated. Can you see how the body might reject them at some point? It's toxic to the body, for heaven's sake!

Finally, a small percentage of us are born with allergies to food substances that our bodies perceive as poison. A common example is a reaction to peanuts. In these cases, we simply can't eat them without risking potentially fatal results. But this condition exceeds sensitivity and rises to the level of a full-blown allergy.

Will I Ever Be Able To Eat Those Foods Again?

For some of us, the answer is, no! For others, as our health improves, we may be able to eat a limited quantity of the foods our bodies are currently sensitive to.

There is an exciting technique we call AACT, or the Advanced Allergy Clearing Technique. This technique helps reduce the hypersensitive reactions for those who are exposed to certain foods, chemicals or metals. Many are able to tolerate exposure with less or no reaction after undergoing treatment, or "clearings," as we refer to them. Miraculous transformations have been experienced with the AACT option.

If you are interested in pursuing the desensitization process, please alert the staff and we will fill you in on both the appropriateness in your situation as well as what to expect.

OK, I've Changed My Diet, But . . . I Feel Hungry All The Time . . . My Energy Level Goes Down . . . I Feel Hyper, Nervous, Angry Or Irritable . . . I Crave Sweets.

Remember, you are making significant changes to the materials (foods) that your body uses to produce energy. Although you're sensitive to some foods and processed foods are nutritionally wanting, your body has adapted in many ways to "stay alive," despite the fact that these adaptations cause problems for you. An extreme example of a body's adaptability to "stay alive" can be demonstrated using the experience of hypothermia.

Hypothermia is a condition caused by exposure to extreme cold for too long. As the body cools down, it reacts by shutting down the blood supply to the extremities, such as fingers and toes, resulting in frostbite. This is simply your body's way of sacrificing what it decides are less important parts compared to organs like the brain, heart and kidneys. The point is that your body makes all kinds of decisions and adapts in ways it sees fit, in order to preserve the best chance of survival. It does this despite that fact that you may suffer in the process.

You may have thought you were getting away with a diet based on sugars and processed food, but sooner or later there is a price to pay. So if after meals you experience a feeling of hunger, reduced energy, nervousness, hyperactivity, anger, irritability or a craving for sweets, then let us know immediately. These are signals that you're running on the wrong blend of fats, proteins and carbohydrates.

As an individual, you need to become aware of the foods you do best with. This includes the ratio of food's basic components: fats, proteins and carbohydrates. Therefore, simple adjustments are often all that are needed to handle the conditions listed in the title of this FAQ. Some may need more good fats like olive, coconut, peanut or sesame oils as well as avocados or fish oils. Others may require more or less protein in the form of red meat, poultry or fish. Finally, others may need more or fewer carbohydrates in the form of fresh fruits and vegetables. Regardless, it is your awareness and communication to us of these clear signals that will enable us to help you find

the right balance. Good things are about
to happen!

Do I Have To Take These Supplements
Forever?

Supplements are just that ~ supplements.
They are used to complete or enhance your
body's lack of wholeness or deficiency. Our
bodies require certain substances that are
essential for healthy function. "Essential" in
the nutritional world means something our
bodies do not produce on their own but is
required to be eaten for normal operation.
Without that something, you lose your
health. If you are like most, this is where
you're at now.

Often I am asked, "Why can't we just
eat more healthy foods instead of using
supplements?" Unfortunately, by the time
you're on a program like ours, your
deficiencies are beyond that which foods
alone can replace. In addition, your digestive
capacities have been compromised in many
cases, requiring nutrition in predigested or
concentrated forms in order to be of any use
to your system.

To complicate things further, so-called
healthy foods don't have the vitamins and

minerals they once did before the persistent application of pesticides, fungicides, herbicides and over-cultivation of the soil. One startling fact is that, to get the same minerals in one cup of spinach that was available in 1945, it would take 45 cups today. Extend this concept to other foods and you can see how foods alone would not re-establish your health.

Therefore, the supplements you take during the fine-tuning and healing phases will, for the most part, not be those you'll require in the maintenance phase. When each and every reflex, i.e. organ or gland, is restored to health, broad-spectrum vitamins, minerals and enzymes are all that are needed to perpetuate good health. For many, this amounts to products like Standard Process's Cyrofood, Calcifood, Multizyme or Zypan and Cardio Plus. This assumes you maintain your newfound eating habits and lifestyle, of course. Bon appétit!

You Said I Was Sensitive To Grains And Sweeteners, But There Are Oats Or Honey In My Supplements.

Standard Process products may contain foods you are supposed to avoid. For instance, you might find one or two containing soy lecithin, oats, wheat or honey. You ask, if you are supposed to avoid them, why do I recommend these products? Simple answer: you tested well for them. But let's take a closer look.

First, when it comes to grains, your sensitivity is to the carbohydrate and/or the protein part of the food, not the germ (as in wheat germ) or the oil (as in wheat germ oil or soy lecithin).

Secondly, the food used in SP products is nearly always organic and not raised with pesticides, herbicides or fungicides. It is processed before rancidity (in the case of oils) or spoilage occurs. It is never stored with preservatives or treated with fumigants. In addition, these supplements are processed using a proprietary method that preserves the balance of vitamins and minerals inherent in the original food. In short, the molecular structure is quite different from that of commercial products found in the marketplace.

You can be assured that when you test well for an SP supplement, it will do its job successfully. Nutrition Response Testing has proven its worth consistently over decades of clinical application. Stick with your program, avoid the foods you are sensitive to, and take your supplements as directed. Your symptoms will improve, and more importantly, your body will begin the process of repairing itself.

Do My Genes Doom Me To Poor Health?

If you believe the media hype, then yes. But the reality is quite different. As I wrote in *The Great Health Heist*, Dr. Francis M Pottenger, Jr. proved through his studies with cats, that food can alter genes. These alterations proved catastrophic, causing cats that ate cooked foods (food a cat would not eat in the wild) to bear offspring that eventually could not survive.

In that book, I didn't mention that Dr. Pottenger's findings were pre-dated by the speculations of Jean-Baptiste Lamarck, a French biologist (1744-1829) who theorized that organisms acquire and pass on adaptations necessary for their survival in a changing environment. Today we call these organisms "genes" and recognize that, when affected by the environment, they change. These altered genes or traits can be passed on to subsequent generations. Dr. Pottenger substantiated Lamarck's theory using food as the environmental factor.

Current science has established that DNA blueprints passed down through genes are not set in concrete at birth. In other words, your genes are not necessarily your destiny!

Environmental influences, including nutrition, stress and emotions, can modify those genes without changing their basic blueprint. And those modifications can be passed on to future generations, as addressed by Bruce Lipton, PhD, in his article, "The Biology of Belief."

A landmark Duke University study was published in the August 1, 2003 issue of *Molecular and Cellular Biology* and highlighted in a "NOVA scienceNOW" segment on PBS in July, 2007. It found that mice with an abnormal gene predisposing them to a yellow-furred coat, obesity, diabetes, cardiovascular disease and cancer, when provided with nutritional supplementation, produced standard lean, brown-furred mice, despite having the abnormal gene. The mice who didn't get the supplements manifested the yellow coat, obesity and a number of the characteristics of diabetes.

In addition, Dr. Dean Ornish, who promotes an extremely low-fat vegetarian diet, reported in his book, *The Spectrum*, on a UCLA study he directed that utilized food to alter genetic markers for prostate cancer. His conclusion: "Although you can't change your genes, you can alter how they are expressed."

Our health is not set in stone. We can take control and make a difference in most circumstances regardless of "the genetic hand" our parents may have dealt us. So wear your genes proudly!

What Is The Science Behind Muscle Testing?

Muscle testing (or applied kinesiology) and Nutrition Response Testing is a relatively new science established in the 1960s through the efforts of Dr. George Goodheart, a highly respected chiropractor, teacher and author who died in 2008. He was a giant in his field and a beacon of truth.

To those practitioners trained to use this modality, nothing uncovers hidden health problems better than muscle testing. To the naysayers, muscle testing is nothing but quackery. Just remember, any change to a customary approach, regardless of the field, is viewed as a challenge to the culturally adopted norm. The best way to change the norm is to show results because, in the end, the results are all that counts. But it never hurts to provide a little information, and so I begin with my own story.

Before I begin, I must share my own initial reaction to muscle testing ~ skepticism. Freddie Ulan, DC, CCN, my mentor and founder of Nutrition Response Testing, loves to embarrass me in front of as many people as he can by describing when we first met.

I had been suffering with poor health for many years and was searching for a solution. One day an acquaintance turned me on to Dr. Ulan. I sat in the back of the room during his workshop, arms folded, in disbelief at what I was witnessing. However, after getting evaluated, I agreed to follow my nutritional healing program to the letter, and within a few weeks I felt better than I had in years.

Back in my clinic, I applied the same method of evaluation to every willing patient and they, too, got great results. At my next workshop with Dr. Ulan, I asked him to teach me everything he knew and he obliged. Before we both knew it, I wrote *The Great Health Heist*, an introduction to Nutrition Response Testing.

So, what is science? What is magic? Are they different?

Just so we understand what we're talking about, the word "science" means "to know" while the definition of "magic" includes terms like "supernatural" or "mysterious."

Arthur C. Clarke, a renowned science visionary and inspiration for the motion picture *2001: A Space Odyssey*, writes in his book, *Profiles of the Future*, that "any sufficiently advanced technology is indistinguishable from magic." In other words, something may seem like magic, but it's really science and technology.

So let's hop into our "way back" machines and return to our childhoods. Can you remember when you first discovered magnetism using a magnet and some iron filings? You placed the filings on a piece of paper or glass and put the magnet underneath. By moving the magnet around, you could move the filings in any direction. In other words, you were demonstrating the nature of electro-magnetic energy and its capacity to penetrate a solid object (the paper or glass).

How does this apply to your physical body? Simple: Your nervous system runs on electricity and is connected to your muscles along with everything else. In short, it is affected by electricity and magnetism and almost any object emitting them.

A dramatic example of this is when a person's heart suddenly stops beating. By receiving a shock of electrical energy, the heart can return to a regular rhythm, beating once again.

Muscle testing simply takes advantage of the electrical properties of all things, especially the subtle emitters of energy like foods, immune challenges, chemicals and metals. If these objects are close enough to the body and strong enough, they will cause a reaction. And this reaction will be reflected in the function of your muscles ~ strengthening or weakening them, for example.

A breakthrough discovery by Dr. Goodheart revealed that this phenomenon could be translated into practical information that, when used by a highly trained practitioner of the healing arts, would lead to a potential strategy to restore normal function to the body.

So, (1) when your practitioner applies pressure on your extended arm while placing his or her hand or a glass container on your body (both being objects that emit a form of electrical energy) and (2) your arm muscle reacts by feeling weaker or stronger, (3) your practitioner is able to design an effective nutritional healing program to restore your body to health and healthy function.

With this knowledge, and your eyes now open to another marvel of Nature, you can more comfortably accept what I believe is the technology of the future.

WHEN THINGS GET TOUGH, THE TOUGH GET GOING

Having second thoughts? The following articles are here to inspire and educate. Knowledge is power so read and re-read for confirmation that you are doing the right thing to improve and maintain your health.

A Celebration Of Life

Can you think of anything more precious than your health? Some may say, my children, my work or my big screen TV. But, depending on how drastically your health is compromised, you may be unable to participate in any activity including the lives of your children.

I have the right to ask this question because over 15 years ago I lost my health. I was so debilitated that simple things including sleeping, working and even thinking were challenges. And I couldn't figure out what had happened. I ate low-fat, lots of whole grains, fruits and vegetables, chicken, fish, some red meat, and I took supplements. Oh, I ate just a little sugar in the form of an occasional ice cream treat or bite of chocolate ~ but just a little. Of course, like most people, I was raised on processed and sugary foods, but I had changed that routine years ago. Yet there I was ~ so sick I needed help getting from bed to chair.

But I refused to allow my condition to get the better of me and eventually found the answer to my question, "What happened to me?" Let me share my discovery.

First, it wasn't an accident or fate that took my health. I allowed it to happen. Maybe not consciously ~ but I put my health in jeopardy. And the same thing is happening or has happened to you.

Second, you have to stop and consider whether what you know and what you do supports your health. Here's a hint: if you are suffering from any symptom or are taking a drug to manage a symptom, then what you know isn't working for you.

So take a look at what we are told to believe is gospel. Media, big business and government agencies have fashioned messages like: "Everyone needs whole grains, fruits, vegetables and low-fat meats." "Cholesterol is bad and chemicals added to foods in the form of colors, preservatives and taste enhancers are safe." "Processed foods (like pasteurized dairy) are just as healthy as raw foods (like raw dairy)." "Prescription drugs are safe." Oh, and everything is measured by blood tests and held to the same standards as if we are all the same.

Yet, since the early 1900s, research consistently questioned this message. But those experts who questioned the corporate trends were suppressed, and the knowledge gained to maintain and restore a person's health using nutrition went underground.

Since what we do depends on what we know, it is no wonder that most statistics about the overall health of Americans lead us in the wrong direction. Especially statistics of chronic degenerative diseases like heart disease, diabetes and obesity. It's time to take a second look. How much longer are you willing to suffer? Aren't you concerned that things may get worse?

My favorite fable is "The Emperor's New Clothes." It is about truth. Out of fear, the emperor's subjects refused to confront him even though he was running around naked. The truth that his new "duds" were simply a figment of his imagination remained unacknowledged until a small, fearless child stepped forward to ask why the emperor was naked. The horrified subjects protested, saying, "The child is wrong. The emperor can't be naked." But truth prevailed.

So we ask, "Amidst all the information bombardment of today's world, what is the truth?" In our case, the truth is plain and simple: **Processed foods, sugar and chemical additives undermine your health and leave you susceptible to illness ~ period!**

Want proof? Here I am some twelve years later, and I'm back with the living-working, playing and teaching. I published my first book, *The Great Health Heist*, and have helped countless people find a personalized nutritional healing program to restore their health like I did mine.

So let's give thanks for our ability to change our mindsets. We have to make some lifestyle changes to see a different result in our health. No matter whether your health concern is preventative or restorative, there is hope. And hope, after all, is the true motivator. Understand that you are in charge if you want to be ~ and be thankful for that. This is what I call "a celebration of life."

Be The Hero of Your Own Life

Who are heroes and why do they inspire us? In ancient Greece, a hero literally was a protector or guardian, the word derived from Hera, the Greek goddess and guardian of marriage. Heroes come through in a clutch, transcending improbable odds. Yet how can an ordinary man or woman hope to be a hero?

In this book I am calling for personal heroics from those who want to be healthy and avoid sickness. Of course, the odds of accomplishing this in a society where bad eating habits and social pressure prevail are nearly impossible.

Consider school, workplace and church gatherings that feature sugary desserts, chip dips and processed foods. Don't forget the holidays and birthdays. And kids want cupcakes and anything sweet. These pressures make it difficult to change our nutritional ways.

BUT this sets the stage for ordinary people like us to rise up and become the heroes of our own lives. So how does a person overcome the odds? First, we have to become aware of our own situation and address it. We have to be open and willing to learn and change. And finally, practice, practice, practice.

This awareness requires an outside, objective view of the current situation. In terms of health, this means a practitioner and a technology that can identify the key pieces of our personal health puzzle, along with a do-able nutrition program that assures we attain our goal.

To Your Good Health!

No matter who you are, what your level of commitment is, or why you've come to a practitioner trained in the nutritional healing arts, there is one common thread: the desire to improve your health. Whether you begin your journey tentatively or flat out, there is a chartable path toward wellness. Your goal is attainable. Like me, you may need to readjust your sights to align your goal with your level of commitment, but always remember, there is hope and we can help.

For additional reading and more information about the topics mentioned here, read my breakthrough book, *The Great Health Heist*.

ABOUT THE AUTHOR
Paul J. Rosen, J.D., L.Ac., EAMP

Paul J. Rosen, J.D., L.Ac., EAMP is a
licensed acupuncturist in Portland, Oregon,
and Vancouver, Washington, where he is
clinic director of AcuNatural Family
Healthcare. A Detroit native, he graduated
from Western Michigan University with a
bachelor's degree in chemistry, mathematics
and philosophy. He holds a law degree from
Indiana University School of Law-
Bloomington and was a trial attorney in
Boston for seven years before deciding to
pursue his interest in alternative healing
methods. He subsequently attended
Emperor's College of Traditional Oriental
Medicine in Santa Monica, California,
graduating with distinction and a master's
degree. Traditional Oriental medicine
includes the disciplines of acupuncture,
herbal medicine, tui na (massage), and
dietary and nutritional therapies among
others.

Following postgraduate work in
Shanghai, China, where he earned a

certificate of achievement, he underwent specialized acupuncture training in Stans, Switzerland. He then studied with Dr. Richard Tan, a master and founder of the "Balance Method" of acupuncture, and presented papers at Dr. Tan's 2002, 2003 and 2004 conferences in San Diego.

Mr. Rosen's most recent achievement is in the field of nutrition where he has won numerous awards from Ulan Nutritional Systems for outstanding contributions in both professional and public education.

His clinic, AcuNatural Family Healthcare, established 18 years ago, is dedicated to health improvement program design as opposed to the conventional "symptom management" model followed by Western Medicine. His studies with Freddie Ulan, DC, CNT, founder of Nutrition Response Testing have enabled that goal, and Dr. Ulan calls on Mr. Rosen to present to other doctors and healthcare practitioners around the country.

His popular call-in radio show called "Health Matters with Paul Rosen" airs regularly in the region. He has appeared on Portland/Vancouver network and community television (KATU-ABC, FVTV) and been interviewed on several radio stations. As an advocate for organic foods and local farmers and farmer's markets, Paul frequently gives public talks and makes himself available as a speaker to interested groups.

Paul Rosen's AcuNatural Family Healthcare clinic is located at 306 East 37th Street in Vancouver, Washington, just across the mighty Columbia River from Portland, Oregon. His mission and that of his enthusiastic clinic team is to provide clients with a true and proven alternative to drugs and surgery. For information on his clinic and practice and current and upcoming events, visit his website: www.AcuNatural.com or call (360) 750-7375. For information about his first book, *The Great Health Heist* and where to purchase it, go to www.TheGreatHealthHeist.com.